CHOOSING THE RIGHT FERTILITY SPECIALIST ISN'T EASY.

Why? Because you are bombarded with confusing medical facts, confusing claims about success, and simply bad information. From super low prices and misleading money-back offers—to unqualified practitioners and unsuccessful, out-of-date methods—how do you ever find a qualified, competent, professional fertility specialist?

You start by reading this patient's guide. In this fact-filled publication, you'll discover our four steps to fertility and how to achieve the ultimate treatment success. Learn about your parenthood options!

Praise for Dr. Palter and his practice from patients:

"Dr. Palter, you are the rock star of fertility specialists!" –MS

"Words cannot begin to express how thankful we are for all you have done for us. During the most challenging time in our lives, you were all there to give us hope and keep our spirits up.... Our happiness and excitement are indescribable.... I would recommend you a million times over." –RN

"Thank you so much for everything you did for us. You all made me feel like I was your only patient. We have highly recommended your office to everyone we know. You're a wonderful group of people...." –CM

Warm, friendly, compassionate, and if you want the job done...! –DKM

Phenomenal staff, excellent bedside manner, always spoke in layman's terms. My family is complete because of Gold Coast. Thank you! –JJM

Get Pregnant Now

A FOUR-STEP PROCESS
TO OVERCOME INFERTILITY

An Expert's Guide
by Board-Certified Reproductive Endocrinologist

STEVEN F. PALTER, MD

Get Pregnant Now
A Four Step Process to Overcome Infertility

Published by
Steven Palter, MD
Gold Coast IVF
246 Crossways Park Drive West
Woodbury, NY 11797

Cover and Interior Design by Dayle Dermatis
Cover Art © mcherevan | Bigstockphoto

ISBN-13: 978-1540770356
ISBN-10: 1540770354

DISCLAIMER/LEGAL NOTICES

Gold Coast IVF does not provide online medical diagnosis, treatment, or prescription of any kind. All information provided in this guide and online is intended to be for general informational purposes only, and is in no way intended to create a physician/patient relationship as defined by state and federal law. This guide is not a substitute for professional medical diagnosis or treatment.

While all attempts have been made to verify information provided in this book, neither the Authors or the Publisher assumes any responsibility for errors, inaccuracies or omissions. Any slights of people or organizations are unintentional. If advice concerning medical or related matters is needed, the services of a qualified professional should be sought.

If you think you may have a medical emergency, immediately call your doctor or dial 911.

TABLE OF CONTENTS

Get Pregnant Now

Introduction

Dear Future Mom or Dad:

Choosing the right fertility specialist isn't easy.

Why? Because you are bombarded with confusing medical facts, confusing claims about success and simply bad information.

From super low prices and misleading money-back offers—to unqualified practitioners and unsuccessful, out of date methods—how do you ever find a qualified, competent, professional fertility specialist?

You start by reading this patient's guide. In this fact-filled publication, you'll discover our four steps to fertility and exactly how to avoid "Seven Deadly Delays" in your treatment for infertility, the "Seven Costly Misconceptions" about fertility treatments, six amazing modern treatment success options, six mistakes to avoid when choosing a fertility specialist, the insider questions to ask a doctor before you start any fertility treatment, and how to achieve the ultimate treatment success—a healthy, happy baby of your own.

I wrote this guide to help you better understand fertility treatments. Now, with this information, you can make an informed, intelligent decision about your needs and options.

And if you have any questions about fertility treatments, causes of infertility, or your options, you're invited to call us at 516-682-8900. We've dedicated our practice to educating patients. We'll be happy to help you in every way.

Best wishes,

Steven F. Palter, MD

Founder, Medical and Scientific Director

Gold Coast IVF Fertility Specialists

Meet Steven F. Palter, MD

Steven F. Palter, MD, is the Founder
and Medical and Scientific Director
of Gold Coast IVF.
He has been a fertility specialist
for over twenty years.

I am a board certified specialist in Ob/Gyn and Reproductive Endocrinology and Infertility and the former Clinical Chief of the Fertility Department at Yale University. I am a professional member of the leading professional societies in my field and an officer of many including the American Society for Reproductive Medicine, The American Association of Gynecologic Laparoscopists, The Society for Reproductive Endocrinology, The Society for Reproductive Surgeons, among many others. My practice is certified by SART, and New York State, and consistently has one of the highest success rates in the nation.

I have been called the expert to the experts in my specialty. I fly to medical conferences around the world to teach physicians the latest in fertility treatments as part of my educational mission. In fact, I am writing this letter to you on a plane, coming home from teaching the leading specialists in Romania.

Why Romania, you ask? Well, the leading fertility specialists there chose me to be the keynote speaker at their first national conference, and then spend a day running their first teaching course. I was made an honorary member of their society and then interviewed on national TV. I consider it an honor to share my knowledge and help patients and doctors realize their fertility dreams… just as I am sharing this same information with you in this free report.

I have dedicated my practice to helping patients to learn about their treatment options and choosing the very best treatments to maximize successful outcomes. This report will give you the tools to make good decisions about your medical care. I and my staff welcome your inquiries and will gladly answer your questions over the telephone.

Gold Coast IVF
Specialists in Fertility Treatments
(516) 682-8900
goldcoastivf.com

Chapter One

*How to Avoid Seven Deadly Delays
in Your Treatment for Infertility*

Delay #1:
Cookie-Cutter Fertility Factory

The wrong treatment on the wrong person at the wrong time. To a hammer everything's a nail…and it is totally wrong to offer the same approach to every patient regardless of their specific diagnoses. Even more surprising is that every place does different tests to make a diagnosis. A 28-year-old woman with irregular cycles should not be doing the same treatment path as a 42-year-old woman who's approaching menopause with irregular cycles!

Delay #2:
Wait and See

Friends, family, and even uninformed doctors tell you to wait and see, just relax, have some wine, give it time.… If you're under 35 and have been having sex without birth control for a year something is wrong and your fertility is much lower than normal. What's more if you are over 35 the time frame drops to 6 months and you have a problem. If there is a problem then waiting just leads to more wasted time and lower chances. Most people don't realize how quickly natural fertility drops with age. Studies have shown for women with no fertility problems the natural chances of conceiving is about 25% between age 20 and 30 years but decreases to below 10% over the age 35.

Delay #3:
But We Haven't Really Been "Trying!"

Patients are often misled by ovulation kits and trying to time the perfect moment to conceive. For them the clock for conception starts ticking with these advanced timing efforts. However fertility experts know that any intercourse without using real birth control has a high chance of conception in a fertile couple. We start the "we've been trying" clock the first day you have unprotected sex—and intercourse with withdrawal still counts.

Did you know the withdrawal method has up to a 40% pregnancy rate? Would anybody tell a high school student who randomly had casual sex "you don't need birth control because withdrawal is safe enough?" Of course not! Withdrawal is not really effective birth control! If it were why would anybody need condoms or the pill?

Delay #4:
Outdated Treatments

Progress is faster in fertility than maybe any other field in medicine. When I teach doctors new techniques I share the old adage that within 5 years everything they do today will be obsolete and if they don't keep pace with these changes then they can't give their patients their best chances.

Everything changes in our field. There are new drugs, new technologies and even new normal ranges of old lab tests! The best fertility expert not only keeps up with all the new research and development, they also know how to personally investigate all the new developments.

Delay #5:
Delay in Diagnosis

Knee jerk jumping to treatments rather than making a diagnosis first. Can you imagine a cancer doctor prescribing chemotherapy before they know what kind of cancer the patient has? Does it make any more sense to start fertility treatment without knowing the root causes?

Delay #6:
Incomplete Diagnosis

They told you they looked for everything, but they only did a surface analysis. What's more confusing is that not all steps to diagnosis are the same! Fertility tests come in many different versions—some more complete and more accurate than others.

Even the most basic x-ray test to see if a woman's tubes are blocked (an HSG) has been shown to be critically dependent on the skill of the specialist doing the test. Imagine the frustration of a couple, who believe the test shows their tubes are open, only to find out months or years later they are really blocked. The x-ray was mistakenly read!

I use the term *causes* of infertility not cause for a reason. Fertility is very complex and in more than half of couples there is more than one reason they can't get pregnant. Why do I spend an hour or more at a new patient consult? Why can't a 20-minute "free initial consult" have real value?

It's because the more carefully the doctor searches the more subtle factors he will find—and each clue uncovered leads to a more specific and accurate personalized treatment. I can count so many cases where a doctor picked the first diagnosis they saw and jumped to treatment that ultimately didn't work because of what they missed! For example, treating a woman with an ovulation problem, without ever checking if her tubes are blocked or if her husband has normal sperm, is a recipe for failure.

Delay #7:
Nobody Has Seen a Problem Like Ours

No matter how unusual your problem, we have seen it before. More than 65% of our patients report that their fear of being weird, strange cases is the number one fear preventing them from picking up the phone and getting the help that they need.

There may be unique combinations and variations, and no two couples are identical, but the basic causes are extremely well known in our modern era of fertility. That's why much of my practice is providing consultations and advice to other doctors. If a general Ob/Gyn finds something they are unfamiliar with, odds are almost certain that as a specialist I've seen it often.

Chapter Two

Seven Costly Misconceptions
About Fertility Treatments

Misconception #1:
It's Going to be Very Expensive and
Not Covered by My Insurance

We are very lucky in NY in that almost every patient has basic fertility benefits that cover all of their testing and most if not all of their treatments.

However to get that coverage, you have to get the appropriate pre-certifications and proceed in the proper fashion. Non-specialists who don't take the time to fight for you won't get you coverage. Over 80% of the people we treat have complete insurance for their treatments no matter what is required. It's frustrating to patients to have to fight over billings and certifications all on their own. We understand how confusing it all is and that's why we employ an insurance coverage specialist to work with you as your advocate and often do all the legwork for you.

There is no reason why finances should prevent you from having a baby. There are additional financing options for those patients that might need them. What many patients don't know is that there is almost always a lower cost and lower tech option that can also lead to success. It just might not be the one the fertility specialist is focusing on.

Misconception #2:
Penny Wise, Pound Foolish

The old saying "If it's too good to be true, it probably is," really applies here. A cut-rate treatment can cost more in time and money than the right treatment at the right time. The actual costs and expenses are very similar between practices. So it just makes sense that if something is being offered at a seemingly too low price, one of two things is happening. Either they are cutting corners or it's just bait and switch.

Just like in construction, if you use cut rate supplies and tools or use untrained labor the project may be cheaper but the results will suffer. I know there are centers that offer special low cost IVF or diagnostic programs but they are *never* the same treatment—they are always mini versions that skip steps to save cost and sacrifice success.

Once again if the half-price version was equally effective no one would ever do the more expensive version. But a bait and switch place will be happy to do a cut rate treatment over and over, ultimately costing the patient more. That's why the real question is not what step A or treatment B costs but what will be the total cost to get to success with each option. A treatment that costs half but offers 1/5th success is no bargain.

Misconception #3:
IVF is Always The Only Answer

This might be an overtreatment for many people, and many people don't need it. IVF is a great treatment that can treat most causes of infertility. For many however it may not be the simplest way to achieve a pregnancy. For almost every cause of infertility there are multiple treatment paths that can lead to a success. Some people want to maximize the chances of a natural pregnancy. Others may want the quickest success possible while others may want to minimize the risk of a multiple pregnancy.

For each diagnosis, I take these factors into account and can help pick a treatment path that meets the couple's unique needs. IVF bypasses most causes of infertility. There is usually the choice of correcting the underlying cause as another option. It's up to you to discuss with your fertility specialist which path most meets your needs.

Misconception #4:
Treatments are Going to Hurt
and Might Put Me in the Hospital

As I said before, there are many causes of infertility. Some of the treatments could be as simple as taking a pill. There are other problems that we can correct permanently as we diagnose them, with no discomfort. There are very few intensive treatments, and treatments that don't involve surgery shouldn't involve hospitalization. When properly done the treatments should not interfere with your normal life.

Misconception #5:
I'll Gain Weight

Well, you might gain weight if you get pregnant! However, the treatments themselves should not cause weight gain. Modern fertility drugs when used properly rarely if ever cause true weight gain. An occasional person might have some minimal temporary water retention (like before your period) that similarly passes on its own.

Nutrition and exercise is so important for general health and fertility as well. I have seen patients so worried about fertility that they stop exercising and start to binge on sweets due to the stress of not being pregnant! These habits can cause weight gain but have nothing to do with fertility treatments.

For this reason we include nutritional and exercise advice for all our patients. Patients who take this path often find they can actually lose weight they have been struggling with, when they start fertility treatments with a whole-health approach.

For other patients weight problems (both too high and too low) may be related to their fertility difficulties. Did you know that both too much and too little weight can cause hormonal problems or that the opposite is also true—hormonal problems can cause weight problems? Ask your fertility specialist about weight, exercise, and nutrition and see if an integrated plan might be right for you.

Misconception #6:
I Might Have to Lose My Job Because Treatment is So Time Consuming

One thing for certain the patients I see are busy. Everybody has a million things on their plates and most moms-to-be are working both in and outside the home- often at more than one job. No one wants to have to choose between paying the bills and having a family- nor should they have to.

A good fertility center will work with you to minimize the interruptions to your schedule from any testing or treatments you need. There are some things that need to be timed to your cycle and others where there is a lot of flexibility possible. The best approach I find is to do all testing together up front for all possible causes and maximize the chance of each and every step working.

Cutting corners and doing only partial testing might seem like it would save time but instead it just makes it more likely the treatments won't work and you'll be filling in the missing tests in 6 months rather than being long pregnant.

A good center should also be able to work with you to understand your work schedule and choose treatments that are least interruptive. Early morning visits once treatments start allow our patients to come in, be seen, and be on their way to work to arrive on time.

Misconception #7: People Who Smoke Get Pregnant All the Time—I Don't Have to Worry That I or My Spouse is a Smoker

It seems that those people who take the worst care of themselves and never want to be pregnant never have trouble getting pregnant (but it's often not true). The effect of smoking and drug use has been extensively studied. If a woman smokes the smoke can directly kill eggs in the ovary and paralyze the little hairs in the fallopian tubes that move sperm and egg together. In fact, women who smoke have the fertility of a woman five years older than they are!

The same things happen in men. Smoking is a common cause of sperm abnormalities. Worse yet, sperm from men who smoke, even when their sperm tests are normal, function much worse than from non-smokers. There is a big difference between people who smoke and have no fertility problems and people with fertility problems who smoke—and find their fertility gets even worse. I think some of my most surprised patients have been the smokers who we helped to quit who got pregnant with no other interventions at all.

Now let's be honest. Quitting smoking is one of the hardest things anyone ever has to do. So if you are having fertility problems and you or your spouse smoke we take a multi-level approach.

First, we set up a plan to raise your chances and add treatments that can solve the problems even if you keep smoking. Next, we offer you help with many different strategies to cut down or quit. That way you are on your way to success from day one, and the more you can cut down the simpler my job is. But either way we are not ignoring the smoking and pretending it's not there. By knowing about it the treatments can be adjusted to maximize the odds at whatever level of smoking you are at.

If you smoke, cutting down or quitting is probably the single biggest change you can make to increase your fertility.

Chapter Three

Six Ways to Fertility Success:
Treatment Options

Treatment #1:
Simple Pills to Treat a Hormonal Problem

Hormonal problems are actually quite common in women. For some women there can be signs of this—most commonly, cycles that are irregular. If a menstrual cycle come at different times each month (more than 5 to 7 days different) there is a good chance fertile eggs are not being released. The same is true if cycles are closer than every 25 days or more than every 35 days. Even more important than your exact cycle length is if there have been any changes.

If your cycle seems different to you—how often or how much—chances are you are correct and something has changed. A good starting point for testing is a home ovulation predictor kit (urine LH kit) available from drugstores. There is no proof that the electronic monitors are any better than the simple urine sticks but name brand kits are more accurate than the non-name discount ones.

One area to be careful is that if the cycles are abnormal the urine kits can give false positives which means the test turns positive but you actually are not ovulating! The opposite can also be true—women with certain hormonal patterns might be perfectly normal but the urine ovulation kits can miss the signal and look like you are not ovulating.

For these reasons the ovulation test kits are only a basic starting test. They can give some idea if the cycle is normal but are not always accurate. To be 100% sure requires special tests from a physician.

I recommend the kits best be used this way at home. For 1-3 months start the ovulation kit on day 10 and test every day. If the kit turns positive research shows you are most fertile if you have sex that night and the next day—that's it! There's no need to try every other day or every day for weeks as you may read (unless you want to for other reasons). If the test is positive around the same days for 2-3 months then you can stop testing and know your fertile time. If this is not enough to achieve pregnancy in the time periods listed above, more specific tests are needed from a specialist.

Irregularities of any hormone system in the body can throw off normal reproduction and make pregnancy harder. One of the most common of these is thyroid disease which frequently has no symptoms at all.

The good news is that even though hormone abnormalities are very common they are among the easiest problems to fix. The testing to identify the problem is simple and easy and usually some simple pills are enough to fix the problem!

If a hormonal problem is present, treatments will usually make women actually feel far better than they felt before. What's more, fixing these problems can significantly improve long term health and well-being beyond fertility and lower the risks of miscarriage when you are pregnant.

Treatment #2:
Fertility Medicine to Enhance a Woman's Ability to Get Pregnant

The first fertility medications I discussed above were to fix hormonal problems when your hormones are abnormal and you are not making an egg as you should. This next group is used to enhance your fertility to even higher levels when you are making eggs normally but other fertility barriers exist.

There are different groups of these medications. Some enhance the development of your egg to ensure the timing of its growth, and to make sure the readiness of the womb to receive it is optimal. This first group of medicines is very simple to take but have limited chances of success.

The next group is more powerful fertility medications that work by having you make more than a single egg each month. You see, at age 35 almost half the eggs a woman makes are not functional and by age forty that number goes up to 80%! So in those cases medications that help you make more than one egg can help raise the odds of a normal sperm and egg meeting.

The same treatment works for similar reasons when sperm counts are low. If only a few sperm are around having more than one egg raises the odds the sperm can find it. What's amazing is this treatment works for most causes of infertility. For example of the tubes where sperm and egg meet are partially damaged or blocked than these drugs again can raise the odds of the tube being able to deliver an egg to the sperm.

Use of these medications is done very differently from center to center. Proper dosage adjustment must be done for each individualized patient. That's because the exact target number of eggs and what does it takes to get there is totally different for every patient! All the subtle details must be taken into account of age, sperm, and other partial factors. Treating too little won't get to a success and treating too much can risk multiple pregnancies unnecessarily.

Treatment #3:
Artificial Insemination—Washing The Sperm and Putting It Inside the Woman With a Little Straw to Give the Sperm a Boost

I remember when artificial insemination with washed sperm was first shown to improve fertility treatments. I was working at Yale and we were surprised that the research showed it was effective for almost every cause of infertility (except blocked tubes).

Sperm are very different in number and function between men. What many people don't know is that even in normal men a majority of sperm don't work! That's one of the reasons why men have to produce millions of sperm at a time. The other reason is that the path to the egg is very very far. For a tiny sperm, swimming and finding the egg would be like walking to California without a map for you and me.

What we learned was amazing. Doctors can actually separate the good sperm from the bad and give them a jump start to fast straight swimming by a washing procedure in the office. This can be done in many different ways and only the best methods truly separate good from bad. Then with a tiny straw the sperm can be placed half-way to the egg in a pain-less 5 minute step. Adding this simple step nearly doubled the chances of success for most fertility treatments!

Treatment #4:
Procedures to Fix Blockages in the Woman's or Man's Reproductive Systems

This is like a plumbing problem—clogged pipes. A man can ejaculate that has little or no sperm in it and similarly women frequently can have blockages in the fallopian tube that can prevent her egg from ever meeting a sperm. The good news is these two problems are among those with the highest success rates when treated correctly.

The worst part of these blockages is…they are silent. They have no symptoms and come on without warning. Often it's a silent infection or inflammation internally that causes it. You might have had a mild stomachache, a fever of 100, or most often no signs at all ….but inside, the passageway for sperm and egg to meet became blocked.

There are two options with blockages. You can fix them with a procedure or you can bypass them with in vitro fertilization (IVF). In either case the key to success begins with identifying the problem correctly.

What's more amazing is the procedures are simpler and less invasive than ever. 30 years ago any procedure required a big incision and major surgery and long recoveries that came with it. Today virtually 100% of the procedures I perform can be done without this invasiveness. For many, no hospitalization is required and procedures can be done painlessly in the office. For those cases where something is done in the hospital, virtually every patient goes home the same day after their "band-aid" procedure.

Treatment #5:
IVF—Putting Egg and Sperm
Together in a Dish

In vitro fertilization (IVF) is now more than 30 years old and it has revolutionized the ability to help couple achieve a healthy pregnancy. I remember when I was young hearing the reports on the news of the birth of the first "test tube baby" Louise Brown and the first US IVF baby Elizabeth Carr shortly thereafter.

One of my favorite recent honors was being invited to sit at dinner with both the UK and American doctors who did these first treatments at the honorary presidential dinner of our national fertility society the ASRM. I was amazed as a child by this incredible treatment that made the impossible seem easy. Now, as a fertility specialist, it was so exciting for me to talk with them about the next stage of developments in our field being developed now.

At first IVF was used only for cases where the problem was with the woman's tubes—where sperm and egg could not meet. In these cases it was a simple bypass to a blocked road. The sperm and egg were made totally normally but the doctors just played dating service and got them to meet in a new location.

Today however IVF has been shown to be one of the most highly successful treatment options for all fertility problems. What's more surprising is we can tailor the treatment to best fit the exact causes in each patient.

30 years ago there were few medication options and ways to follow the eggs. Today we have so many new options that are simpler and more convenient. For example we can now use a noninvasive ultrasound to take pictures of the developing eggs and know when they are perfectly ready to meet the sperm as opposed to guessing or using urine tests like in the past.

IVF success rates have climbed dramatically over the past decades. The first pioneers had less than a 1% chance of success. When I started my training as a fellow at Yale success rates were around 15%. I am so happy that I've been able to double that rate TWICE since I opened my center in NY.

Some patients tell me they are too scared to consider IVF because they see it as the last resort…and what would they do if it did not work? I tell them it's a very effective treatment and the key is matching them to what treatments they truly NEED. If they need IVF, then delaying that step only delays their likely success. If IVF isn't their best option then they should consider one of the simpler treatments first.

Another important discussion I have with my patients is the time needed to get to their pregnancy. This is an area where IVF has some advantages over other treatments. For example for some patients IVF could have a 4-5 times higher chance of pregnancy in a single month than another option. So while both paths can lead to success, the downside of the simplest treatment is it might take 6 months instead of one.

Now if the couple has not been trying too long, are very young, or don't feel a sense of urgency the slow simple path might be very attractive. For couple in their late 30's or who have been trying for many years, or who just don't want to face the chance of another period coming then IVF will be more attractive.

Treatment #6:
Amazing Recent Options for IVF—
Sex Selection And Genetic Health Testing

In standard IVF we work to get the sperm and egg together and to achieve a pregnancy. There are two seldom discussed options that are very important for some parents-to-be. Both of these involve taking the 3 day old embryo when it's just 6-8 cells and doing genetic testing on just one of those cells.

The first is sex selection commonly used for what is called "family balancing". I have seen couples who develop infertility later in their relationship who already have children. In some cases they have a beautiful boy or girl and have been struggling for their second child and don't plan more children after that and dream of balancing their family with one child of each sex. In other cases the family may have 2 or 3 children of the same sex before they develop their infertility.

In both of these cases we can help them overcome their infertility and balance their family at the same time. There are even some couples who choose this treatment who don't have fertility problems. Every couple is different when it comes to deciding if balancing their families matters a little a lot or not at all.

The second way this genetic testing is used is to help prevent genetic illnesses or miscarriages. If a couple carries a genetic disease, in the past they would have to take the huge risk of trying to get pregnant and if the child had the disease either it would not survive or they might choose termination.

Today if we know the couple is at risk (and we can actually do a lot to determine if risks occur for people who have no such family history) we can determine which embryos are healthy and which are not and prevent a pregnancy that would not survive. We can do the same testing for the most common forms of miscarriage and down's syndrome as well.

Chapter Four

*Six Mistakes to Avoid When
Choosing a Fertility Specialist*

Mistake #1:
Assuming All Fertility Doctors Are the Same

Fertility doctors are not all the same. The most fundamental differences are related to training, attitude, and how hard they work to keep up with what's new. Having been the Clinical Chief of the Fertility Department at Yale where I ran the training fellowship, I am well aware of the huge differences in skills learned at the different programs. I remember very clearly when I myself applied for my fellowship.

I loved all the different parts of the fertility field. These included solving hormonal problems, IVF, male fertility treatments, and amazing keyhole laser microsurgery. However, I was surprised to see some training programs that excelled at only one or two of the facets of the specialty.

One of the reasons I chose Yale was because the program there insisted on fellows learning all the different parts of the specialty with equal expertise—because they were all equally important. The first mistake is a facility that offers just one solution, just one path to parenthood. If everyone in the waiting room is doing the exact same treatment something is wrong. There is no single treatment option that is always best for all patients.

The physician's attitude once they leave their training is also crucial to your success and how pleasant or unpleasant the treatment process will be for you. Here is where physicians are separated into those that probe for causes of fertility problems vs. those that look on the surface. Those that work with you to educate and make you feel comfortable with the process vs. those that just seem bothered by your questions. Those that reevaluate each step of treatment vs. those that only make changes when you ask them to.

The desire to keep up to date is another vital difference between physicians. I am continually amazed at how fast advances come in our field. I've learned never to take any treatment or step for granted and know every step can and will be improved. It's vital for physicians to go to the major medical meetings and keep up by reading the latest medical research.

In the lecture I gave in Romania I finished by telling the doctors everything you do today will be obsolete and replaced within the next five years—and here's why you should be excited by what's better coming soon rather than scared of what going to be replaced!

Mistake #2:
Too Many Cooks Spoil The Broth—
Factory Fertility

When I worked at the University there were 7 physicians and more than half a dozen fellows, not to mention the huge staff of nurses and support staff. Some of the biggest frustrations I and patients had came from the changes in who was making the decisions on any given day. If there is not a major focus on exact consistency of all treatment (which rarely occurs) the end result becomes one of details getting lost and inconsistency in treatment.

I believe in order to be truly excellent in caring for a fertility patient, the person who makes the treatment decision each and every day needs to know all the important details of the couple.

That includes their normal and abnormal tests, the past attempts at treatment that did not work no matter where they were done, their preference and priorities, and each step of how they responded to past treatments.

If you are in the middle of treatment and find you need to explain who you are or what your fertility problem is to the doctor of the day there is no way they can know all the details required to perfect your treatments. The end result sadly is often the same mistakes being made over and over again.

Mistake #3:
Places That Don't Offer All the Treatments That Are Available Today

I've seen this happen two ways. The most common is the "I only have one tool" approach. You know the saying, if you only have a hammer, all the world's problems look like nails.

Part of this might be training that focused on only parts of our specialty and part might be doctors who rely on only a subset of treatments. Some treatment options are much simpler for the doctor (not the patient) and some sadly to say are more profitable for the doctor than others. At the best centers these two factors should never shape your treatment plan.

One good question to ask is "are there other treatment options for my problem that you yourself don't do that you could refer me to another doctor for?" I always discuss all the treatment options with my patients and help them rank their top to bottom choice before we even check into insurance coverage.

The second reason why some treatments might not be offered is if the doctor does not keep up with all the cutting edge developments in our field. In general, if someone is practicing the same way he did five years ago then he's likely to be getting out of date!

While this is hard for patients to know, one clue is asking questions about what update meetings and readings the specialist routinely participates in.

Mistake #4:
Untrained "Specialists"—
The So-Called Specialist Who Isn't

To be board certified as a fertility specialist, a doctor must be first board certified in obstetrics and gynecology, and then board certified in reproductive endocrinology and infertility as well. This requires both training in ob/gyn and an approved fertility fellowship, as well as passing certifying examinations.

Any general ob/gyn can call themselves a fertility special-ist and some do very good work. But in general, they won't perform all the most advanced treatments certain patients may require or have experience with more unusual cases. They cannot call themselves reproductive endocrinologists. There is no official specialty for reproductive immunology although this term may be used by some doctors.

The Society for Reproductive Endocrinology (part of the American Fertility Society) recommends you ask what your fertility doctor's training is and if they are board certified fer-tility specialists. These certifications must be renewed each year and show a commitment to ongoing review licensure and quality of care.

Mistake #5:
Picking Location Over Quality

You need the best, not the closest. Treatment that doesn't work is much less convenient in the long run. If you ask most doctors or nurses how they find a specialist to solve a complex medical problem in their family what they will tell you is they start off by finding the best specialist they possibly can reach.

Starting the search by zip code is backwards. Maybe you'll save 15-60 minutes driving to your first visit but imagine the difference between an integrated treatment plan that succeeds with half the office visits and in half the months of trying vs. the place next door wasting time on unnecessary visits and ineffective treatments.

What's more, spread out places with a lot of different locations cannot give you personalized, individualized treatment. They are going to be too spread out with remote teams making decisions about patients they have never seen.

Mistake #6:
Assuming Your Hopes and Desires, Preferences and Fears Cannot Be Part of The Treatment Decision

In other words, assuming the doctor just tells you what to do and that you have no choices. There is almost always more than one treatment option and the following factors should be addressed by your specialist to individualize your treatment choice path.

1. How quickly do you feel you need to ensure a success ? 3-months? 6-months? Or one- year?
2. Do you want to do as little as possible and conceive the most naturally or does the level of high-tech treatment not matter to you?
3. Do you want to avoid any invasive treatments or tests?
4. Do you have religious or cultural limitations on testing or treatments?
5. Could you accept a pregnancy that was twins?
6. How many children more do you want to have? One more or several?

Chapter Five

Four Steps to Get Pregnant Now: A Strategy to Achieve Success Today

These steps are a summary of all the information you learned here in this guide. Here is how you apply everything you learned to make an action plan to achieve your goals.

Step #1:
Make a Commitment to Yourself to
Get the Help You Need, as Soon as You Can

The clock is ticking, and time will run out faster than you would want to believe. If you do need help, it is important for you to find the right specialist, the way we discuss here in the guide.

Check the credentials of potential fertility specialists you might see. At your first visit see if they see you as a partner in deciding which treatment path is best for you. See if they want to hunt for the cause of the problem before they choose a treatment option for you.

Step #2:
List Your Objectives

Do you want to just go to the first doctor you find? Or do you want to explore the reasons for your infertility and the best centers to treat your specific causes of infertility? Are you using price or value as your guide for making important medical decisions about your fertility and health?

Find the right expert to help you chart your pathway to pregnancy.

Step #3:
Ask Questions

The way you learn about a fertility center is to ask specific questions and listen carefully to the answers. Here are eight tough questions to ask a fertility specialist before you choose a doctor for treatment:

1. What fertility treatments do you recommend and why?
2. What kind of diagnostic methods do you use?
3. What is the success rate for the treatment that you recommend?
4. How soon should I get this treatment?
5. What training have you had in fertility and where?
6. Are you a member of ASRM, SART, and the AAGL (our biggest fertility IVF and surgical professional societies)? Do you attend these meetings each year? How often do you teach other doctors at these meetings and have you won any awards in the last few years?
7. Are you board certified by the American Board of Ob Gyn as both an Ob/Gyn AND a Reproductive Endocrinologist /Fertility Specialist? Is your certification current?
8. Is your lab certified?

Step #4:
Once You're Satisfied That You're Working With a Well-Trained, Professional Fertility Specialist, Sit Down for a Consultation and Ask for a Review of Your Condition and a Recommended Course of Treatment

This should be comprehensive and involve a history of you and your partner and exam and often an ultrasound or other tests. The process should take around an hour.

Once your consultation is complete, you should have a clear diagnosis of what's preventing you from becoming pregnant. Your diagnosis or diagnoses should make sense to you based on everything that has happened in your fertility history. The diagnosis should include all factors and not be based on the first, most obvious cause.

Your treatment should be based on the diagnosis, and should be re-evaluated every single month that you are not pregnant. You should reassess with your doctor exactly why it didn't work.

Every unsuccessful attempt should shed new light on your situation, lead to a modification to your plan, and represent a step closer to ultimate success.

Chapter Six

Contact Us

By following these four steps, you'll gain all the information you need to make an informed, intelligent decision about your fertility treatment. You deserve the best, most experienced and compassionate care.

At Gold Coast IVF, we have a passion for empowering our patients and giving them every medical advantage to achieve ultimate success. We'd be happy to meet with you and guide you through our specialized Comprehensive Fertility Audit™ which identifies exactly what your barriers to fertility are and enables us to develop your Roadmap to Success™ - an individualized plan to achieve your pregnancy in a way that meets your needs, concerns, and time frame.

Call us at (516) 682-8900 to schedule our meeting and take the next step to make your family dreams come true.

About the Author

Dr. Steven Palter: GOLD COAST IVF

Dr. Steven Palter is the Founder and Medical and Scientific Director of Gold Coast IVF in Woodbury, NY. For over 20 years, he has dedicated his career to making the dreams of infertile couples come true and is internationally recognized as a leader in the field of fertility treatment. He has treated patients from all over the world, and his work is frequently featured in the press, including Nature, CBS News, and the New York Times. The leading news program *20/20* featured Dr. Palter and his work in a special segment, as did *National Geographic*.

Dr. Palter's center has achieved extraordinary results for his patients, and reports among the highest success rates in the United States.

CLINICAL RESEARCHER
AND MEDICAL INNOVATOR

As a member of the Yale faculty, Dr. Palter was Clinical Chief of Reproductive Endocrinology and the Founder and Director of many additional programs including the Advanced Endoscopy Fellowship and the Yale Oncofertility Program. He has served as the first-ever Editor for Video and New Media for the leading fertility journal, Fertility and Sterility of the American Society of Reproductive Medicine, ASRM. He has also served on the ASRM Board of Directors, the Society of Reproductive Endocrinology, and the Society for Reproductive Surgery.

Dr. Palter has also served on the Board of Directors of the leading minimally invasive surgery society in the world, the AAGL. Dr. Palter founded and is the Program Director for the International Center of Excellence Program in Minimally Invasive Gynecologic Surgery. Dr. Palter's passion for technological innovations is well known, and he has been honored to speak as Plenary and Keynote Speaker for both ASRM and AAGL more than any other physician.

He is well known for cutting-edge technological developments and collaborations with innovators from outside medicine. He performed the world's first HD and 4K surgeries and has developed award-winning techniques to visualize disease and embryo details invisible to the naked eye. Dr. Palter is a Sony HD luminary and an advisor to Red Digital Cinema.

He has been awarded international prizes for his research over six times, and is a top ranked speaker in his field. The leading medical organizations have sought Dr. Palter as an invited Professor and lecturer, including Yale University, the Cleveland Clinic, and more than 20 other universities and national fertility/surgical societies.

MEDICAL THOUGHT LEADER AND EDUCATOR

Dr. Palter's expertise extends beyond new developments in his field. He is also a noted expert in using technological advances in other industries to bridge gaps in medical education, surgical innovations, and transformation of medical literature.

Dr. Palter's practice and research both focus on infertility and advanced endoscopy and he serves as reviewer for many journals. He is the recipient of numerous research grants, taught over 100 invited lectureships/courses, has over 80 publications and abstracts, mentored trainees from over a dozen nations, and been invited to perform laparoscopic and hysteroscopic surgery around the world.

He is also the developer of the Lodestone platform for online education and collaboration. Over forty university departments use this system to educate their fellows, present new research, and reach out to patients, including Harvard,

University of Pennsylvania, Stanford, UCLA, the Cleveland Clinic, and the NIH.

Dr. Palter is also passionate about educating the next generation of medical practitioners, inventors, and Nobel Prize winners. In addition to his surgical students and the fellows he mentors through his Lodestone online education platform, Dr. Palter recently spoke to thousands of high school students and educators at the National Academy of Future Physicians conference, sharing the stage with such luminaries as Craig Ventner and Peter Diamandis. Dr. Palter organized and moderated a ground-breaking live telesurgery session for high school students, the first one ever presented.

HOMETOWN DOCTOR

Above all, however, Dr. Palter values the gift of his own family. He married his high school sweetheart, has three boys, and moved back to his hometown after completing his training and his tenure as Clinical Chief at Yale. He is devoted to bringing his happiness to every person on the journey to parenthood.

For more information, please contact Dr. Palter at

Gold Coast IVF
246 Crossways Park Drive West
Woodbury, NY 11791
(516) 682-8900
palter@gcivf.com
www.goldcoastivf.com